INTRODUCTION

Dry January is a public health campaign encouraging individuals to abstain from alcohol for January, especially practiced in the United Kingdom, France, and Switzerland.

The campaign, as a former entity, seems, by all accounts, to be moderately recent, being portrayed as having "jumped up as of late" even in 2014. However, the Finnish government had launched a campaign called Sober January in 1942 as a feature of its war effort. The expression "Dry January" was registered as a brand name by the charity Alcohol Concern in mid-2014; the first-ever Dry January campaign by Alcohol Concern happened in January 2013. In the lead-up to the January 2015 campaign, unexpectedly Alcohol Concern partnered with Public Health England.

As indicated by Alcohol Concern in January 2014, which started the campaign, more than 17,000 Britons quit drinking for that month. While there is controversy regarding the viability and advantages of the practice, a 2014 overview by the University of Sussex found that a half year following January 2014, out of 900 studied participants in the custom, 72% had "held hurtful drinking scenes down" and 4% were yet not drinking.

Dry January, as in dumping alcohol in the first month of the new year, is a yearly custom or tradition for many individuals. For a few, a fresh new year's resolution needs to drink less, while others guarantee it is an approach to "detox" from excessive drinking over the special seasons or holiday.

Partaking in Dry January may be particularly appealing after the isolation, stress, and forlornness of 2020. Many individuals report drinking more than expected, and proof proposes individuals are using alcohol to assist adapt to stress brought about by the pandemic. Maybe you are one of them and might want to commence 2021 by purposefully not utilizing alcohol to cope for a while.

Many people are not ordinarily devotees of fad diets or gimmicky health changes that may not be manageable for the long stretch. That is because any kind of deprivation with an expiry date watches out for not have a lot of advantages once it is over (if by any means).

However, to the extent health patterns go, Dry January appears to be quite innocuous—indeed, requiring a one-month rest from drinking could do truly incredible things for your well-being. You will capitalize on Dry January, notwithstanding, if you utilize the month as an opportunity to reassess (and potentially change) your drinking propensities and relationship with alcohol after the month is up—instead of a permit to drink as much as you need the remainder of the year.

CHAPTER ONE

Dry January Benefits-Your General Health May Improve.
It is not news to anybody that inordinate drinking and binge drinking prompt a few negative health effects, including hypertension and elevated cholesterol, women's health expert Jennifer Wider, M.D., advises women that specializes in health, beauty, and style.

Inordinate drinking additionally debilitates your sleeping pattern and increase the risk for specific diseases, including breast cancer, heart disease, stroke, and liver problems, she says. (Peruse more about the negative health effects of drinking an excessive amount of alcohol over the short and long term).

Even though going without alcohol for one month will not treat or prevent long term health problems, it probably could not hurt taking everything into account. In as much we do not know precisely what enduring effect (assuming any) Dry January will have on your health, it is reasonable to assume that abstaining from drinking is for the most part useful for your general health—if you do not use this hiatus to drink vigorously during the remaining 11 months of the year.

With regards to your liver, for example, we do realize that alcohol puts metabolic stress on the liver and that about half of all liver sickness deaths are from alcoholic liver disease, says Koob. Given the expanding rate of millennials dying from alcohol-related liver diseases, relaxing this imperative organ surely is not the most exceedingly terrible thought.

And keeping in mind that there are not some enormous, thorough investigations on the health effects of momentary restraint, there is some proof that one month off drinking can prompt health benefits, at any rate temporarily and in the near-term.

In one observational investigation, published in the British Medical Journal in 2018, researchers tracked 94 healthy moderate-to-heavy drinkers who avoided alcohol for one month and discovered upgrades in different health markers like blood pressure, liver function tests, insulin resistance, and molecules that assume a job in cancer growth.

The authors call attention to, notwithstanding, that these momentary discoveries do not set up enduring health effects from one month of forbearance, and that one month off drinking does not refresh your liver.)

At that point, there is likewise the way that an ever-increasing number of women are winding up in the emergency room from alcohol-related causes, which implies that scaling back alcohol (or removing it totally) may bring down your risk of an intense health emergency also.

2. You'll Perceive How Your Body Feels Without Booze.

The greatest advantage is realizing where your body is comparable to alcohol and what you want your relationship with it to be says Koob. If, for example, you have been feeling not your best of late and you speculate that your regular (or excessive) drinking propensities may be adding to that, it could be useful to perceive how you are feeling (intellectually, physically, socially, and so on) when you do not have alcohol for a month.

For certain individuals, it tends to be an incredible method to hit the reset button and get their frameworks in the groove again, New York-based registered dietitian Jessica Cording, M.S., R.D., advises. It is not an ill-conceived notion, particularly if you are attempting to cut down on your drinking.

3. You Might Sleep Better And Feel More Invigorated.

Dry January may likewise be useful for your sleep and energy levels, which thusly have their constructive outcomes. It might help you feel even more composed and experience better sleep alongside ordinary digestion-Cording says. This can help you feel more vigorous and remain inspired to get in your workouts and stick to overall healthy eating propensities.

What is more, the sheer reality that you are not keeping awake until late drinking most nights can prompt sleeping more and skipping workouts less? The entirety of that can affect how productive you are, the manner, and how focused at work you are, and how you feel, by and large, says Koob—a sort of snowball impact.

4. Your Immune Framework Might Be In Better Shape.

Drinking an excess of alcohol can debilitate your immune framework, as indicated by the NIAAA. As per Koob, being inebriated can intensely suppress immune function, making you more vulnerable to pathogens, while constant drinking can prompt inflammatory reactions all through the body.

Indeed, even one night of heavy drinking can hinder your ability to ward off infections up to 24 hours after, per the NIAAA. (And keep in mind that being more helpless against becoming ill is never acceptable, it is particularly hazardous during the COVID-19 pandemic, as Kenneth Leonard, Ph.D., director of Clinical and Research Institute on Addictions at SUNY University at Buffalo, disclosed to American online magazine for women that specializes in health, beauty, and style recently.)

Additionally, those positive conduct transforms we referenced above—like eating healthfully, getting enough sleep, and exercising regularly—are healthy propensities that can support your immune framework in the long haul, as SELF has recently revealed.

5. If Weight Loss Is Your Goal Scaling
Back On Drinking May Help.

To start with, note that cutting calories with weight loss as an objective is not the correct decision for everybody, because the relationship between weight and health is more muddled greater and weight-loss diets generally do not work in the long term.

In case you are having several drinks on weekly basis, one after-effect of Dry January could be a decline in your caloric intake, since a standard drink typically has around 150 calories, says Koob. Furthermore, in contrast to, say, removing a certain nutrition type or limiting caloric intake from food, cutting alcohol will not settle on any of the fuel and supplements your body needs to feel satisfied and nourished.

"Alcohol contributes calories but doesn't cause us to feel more fulfilled—it regularly amps up an appetite," Cording clarifies. Furthermore, its ability to debilitate your judgment may lead you to settle on imprudent food choices that sound extraordinary at the time—like requesting enough takeout for three, for instance —but can cause you to eat way past the purpose of fullness and/ or potentially feel kinda awful the following day. (If you have ever experienced a sugar hangover and an alcohol hangover simultaneously, for example, you precisely know the thing we are discussing.)

6. You Might Reevaluate Your Relationship With Alcohol.

When Dry January is over, check-in with yourself to perceive how the experiment went and what that may mean for your drinking propensities going forward. Here are the sorts of inquiries you might pose to yourself: Do you feel improved? Healthier? Are you More productive? More profitable? Not as different as you thought you might. Have your sleep, mood, or exercise pattern changed? Have you saved money?

Do you have a freshly discovered gratefulness for the ritual of having a glass of red with dinner? Possibly you have discovered that you are more energized without all those hangovers, or you are less anxious following a night of drinking. Or on the other hand, hey—perhaps you have discovered that you essentially feel the equivalent and simply miss the social parts of drinking with friends over a Zoom happy hour. These are useful takeaways to consider after your experiment.

WHAT DRY JANUARY MIGHT LOOK LIKE TO YOU

As a rule, the advantages of Dry January will rely upon what your baseline drinking practices are, George F. Koob, Ph.D., director of the National Institute on Alcohol Abuse and Alcoholism (NIAAA), advises by women that specializes in health, beauty, and style.

Somebody who drinks every so often presumably will not see as a very remarkable contrast as somebody who has four or five drinks in one night— a few nights per week. Thus, for our purposes, we should accept that we are discussing somebody who drinks more than what is considered "moderate," which relies upon who is defining "moderate."

The NIAAA utilizes the USDA Dietary Guideline to characterize moderate drinking as up to one drink for each day for women and two drinks per day for men. Heavy drinking, as indicated by the NIAAA, implies consuming multiple more than 3 drinks in a day for women or more than 4 drinks for men.

The Substance Abuse and Mental Health Service Administration (SAMHSA) has a somewhat extraordinary definition, depicting heavy alcohol use as binge drinking (at least four drinks for women and at least five drinks for men on a similar event) on at least five days in the past month, the NIAAA clarifies. So, if your drinking propensities are closer to "weighty" than "moderate," per these rules, remember that this change might be somewhat harder for you than for another person.

You ought to likewise be cautious—and possibly give your doctor a heads up—before suddenly halting drinking if you have been drinking heavily.

At whatever point you go without any weaning period after intensely drinking consistently, it is conceivable to experience mild-to-moderate side effects or symptoms of alcohol withdrawal that vibe like an awful, broadened hangover, for example, anxiety, irritability, nausea, fatigue, headache, and shakiness, as indicated by the United State of America National Library of Medicine.

Individuals with a background marked by heavy drinking might be in danger of a severe type of alcohol withdrawal, the U.S. National Library of Medicine clarifies, which is the reason alcohol-dependent people frequently need medical support to quit drinking.

And in case you are somebody with a higher risk of seizures, you need to connect with your doctor and be particularly mindful. The vast majority will consider it as a hangover, but if you are inclined to seizures or are on seizure medication, unexpectedly halting liquor could trigger a seizure, says Koob.

BOTTOM LINE

Dry January can have some incredible health advantages if you go about it the correct way.

It does not hurt to take an interest in Dry January. But you will receive the most health rewards if you consider it a springboard to revisit your overall relationship with alcohol. Once more, jettisoning alcohol for a month and afterward continuing your usual drinking propensities will not do much for your long-term health if you try to overdo it when it is not Dry January.

This is certainly not an extraordinary pattern: binge/decline, binge/abstain-Dr. Wider extensive says. Much the same as other substances, alcohol in overabundance has health consequences, whether you go dry for a month. That is the reason she says your overall health should be a moderate drinker all in all—as opposed to going from one extreme to the next.

Once Dry January is over, use what you have learned about your relationship to drinking to inform how you approach it pushing forward. Learn from the experience, says Koob. What is your relationship with alcohol, and where would you like to be? - Cording concurs. This is an incredible chance to consider what a reasonable measure of alcohol is for your way of life-she says. Consider how to fit it in such a way that feels balanced.

Something more to remember as you wrap up Dry January: Your resistance to alcohol's effects will regularly be lower following a month without drinking, Koob says, so be mindful so as not to try too hard the first time when you have a drink once more.

THOMAS COLVIN

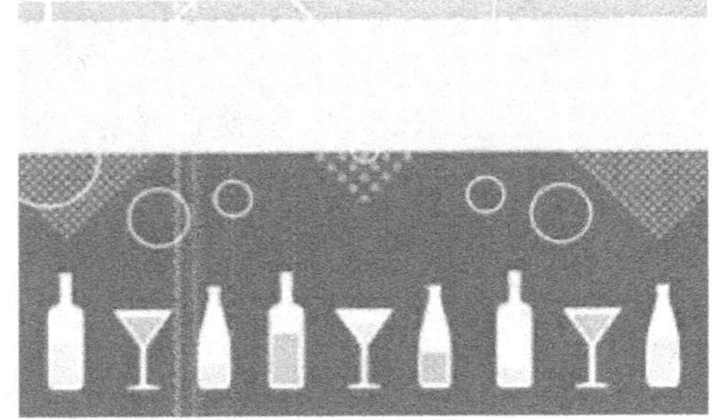

CHAPTER TWO

10 HINTS AND TIPS FOR A BRILLIANT DRY JANUARY

If a month is spent without alcohol automatically, that will do wonders for your health - here we offer a few clues and tips to make it the most ideal experience for January and beyond!

1. REMIND YOURSELF OF YOUR MOTIVATIONS

On what ground would you say you are doing this? Make a rundown of the relative multitude of things you want to gain. At that point rank them in order of significance - give them a score out of 10. Investigate your rundown and spotlight on how you will accomplish all these magnificent things.

Truly, you will likely set aside a touch of money yet what has truly roused you to take this journey? In what manner will you feel when you succeed? Put everything down in writing and stick it someplace noticeable as an update consistently. This will help you pay attention to your Dry January and continue onward if circumstances become difficult.

2. TELL PEOPLE.

It very well may be enticing to keep quiet about your Dry January, particularly in case you are worried you will not endure the month, but telling others is a decent method to keep you on target. Post your goal via social media. In case you are going out, let your people know ahead of time that you will not drink. You might find that lots of others are doing Dry January as well!

3. Decide A Plan for Situations where Alcohol Is On Offer.

You are likely going to be welcomed someplace where there will be alcohol on offer at some point in January, so you should be prepared. Choosing already the thing you will do in those circumstances will truly help you when the opportunity arrives.

Regardless of whether it is adhering to alcohol-free alternatives options (that resemble the genuine deal – if your local does not stock alcohol-free beer and wine you could attempt a soda and lime), recommending everybody buys their drinks or practicing saying no, ensure you have an arrangement good to go!

4. PRACTICE SAYING NO

You do not have to legitimize your choice to remain dry in January obviously, but now and again it assists with having an instant explanation if somebody gets pushy and demands you go along with them in a drink. Perhaps "I'm doing Dry January" won't generally be your go-to reason, so what else would work for you? I am driving/caring for my mental health/running a virtual long-distance race tomorrow/taking care of the children in the morning? Simply ensure if somebody offers you a drink unexpectedly, you have your answer prepared. It is good, so a lot simpler than attempting to think about an explanation when somebody calls you out. If you remain firm, individuals are more averse to attempt to persuade you to alter your perspective.

5. PLAN SOME ACTIVITIES TO ANTICIPATE.

After the year we have had, goodness realizes we could all do with something to anticipate. Arranging some pleasant activities during January will make it a ton better and give you a little jolt of energy if 2021 tosses us more curves.

Also, not drinking will save you money – so utilize some of it to treat yourself! Only a couple of potential activities include going on a stroll with a friend, attending a virtual life drawing class, teaching yourself a new instrument, attempting an alternate takeaway eatery, or preparing yourself an intricate feast each week, going on a road trip somewhere, getting yourself some truly extravagant tea/espresso/hot chocolate/soft drinks... and most, if not all, of these activities, should be possible even with COVID-19 restriction in place!

Showing yourself that you need not bother with alcohol to have some good times will stand you in splendid stead going ahead.

6. BE READY FOR MISTAKES/SLIP-UPS

Being ready for mistakes/Slip-Ups is a smart thought. Having a drink should not be the apocalypse – or even the finish of your dry month. It just relies upon your mentality and how you come back from it.

Try not to whip yourself about any mistakes/slip-ups. Simply consider why it happened – what made it troublesome not to drink? Could there be something you can do next time to stop you from drinking? That way, if a similar circumstance comes up once more, you will be more ready. That, in turn, will assist you with reinforcing what we like to call your 'drink-refusal aptitudes', and that will make scaling back after January if you want to a doddle.

7. KEEP A DIARY

Record what is going on, what is extraordinary, what is better each day. You can glance back at past sections and see exactly how far you have come. Making time each day, even only a few minutes, to help yourself to remember your Dry January journey will truly assist you with owning it as far as possible. Why not blog about your Dry January encounters? This might be something to rouse your colleagues or family or just to keep you considering your Dry January adventure.

8. TELEPHONE A FRIEND

Doing Dry January with a friend can have a significant effect. You can inspire and encourage each other and have somebody to go to if it gets tough. Better still, get the entire group included! Feeling propelled by the thing others are accomplishing and not having any desire to let others down are both incredible approaches to remain committed. Individuals who get together with a friend are significantly more liable to succeed. If it is a friend, you are serious with, it is even far and away superior!

9. CONSIDER WHY YOU DRINK AND MAKE A SWITCH.

What are the things that make you extremely want a drink? For some individuals, the triggers can be categorized as one of the four classes - Social Occasions, Treats, Negative Feelings, or Defenses Down. These can be internal (considerations, emotions, or sensations) or external (things going on around you). Realizing your triggers can truly assist you with getting ready for enticing occasions and work out certain things you can do all things considered. For instance, if you drink because you are stressed, might you be able to give going a shot a stroll instead?

10. REQUEST HELP IF YOU NEED IT.

You might detect that Dry January is harder than you suspected, and that is alright. You could have a go at having a Drier January instead, and utilize the Try Dry app to set some objectives. In case you are thinking that it is tough, do not battle through wretchedly. Instead, converse with somebody. That might be your loved ones, or it very well may be your GP or local alcohol services, so be mindful so as not to overdo it the first time when you have a drink once more.

CHAPTER THREE

HOW TO DO DRY JANUARY DURING CONVID-19

This January will be quite extraordinary - so here are some top tips for taking on a dry month during CONVID-19.

Last year has been somewhat of an odd one, most definitely. A considerable lot of us have spent it stressed, anxious, and worried, and a few of us might have developed drinking propensities we would prefer to break. Dry January offers the ideal occasion to do exactly that.

"However, how?" we hear you inquire. Indeed, Dry January is the ideal possibility for a break. A complete reset. Four weeks to take a stab at something new. Reclaim your mornings. Unwind with a bath, not a bottle. Throw off the 2020 funk and jump into a new hobby with energy. It is not tied in with surrendering something, but rather about getting something back. Your time, your energy, your fun, your freedom. Get your YOU back.

Be that as it may, how would you take on a Dry January is among the ongoing CONVID-19 vulnerability, with stress levels still so high? Here is a portion of our top tips, highlighting advice from individuals who have been moderating or alcohol-free throughout the pandemic.

1. PREPARATION IS KEY.

Preparation is critical. There will be occasions when you will need alcohol, so choose ahead of time how you will manage these cravings. Permit yourself some chocolate or other treat in the first few days which are the hardest, the longer you go the simpler it gets.

Bill

Try not to have alcohol in the house, attempt heaps of alcohol-free beer/cocktail alternatives, use the Attempt Dry app to track dry days, read however much as could be expected (from dependable sources) about how alcohol influences our body and mind, discover something to do to take your mind off alcohol, be interested and try things out without judging yourself.

The prospect of taking on a Dry January currently may feel hard. But the stunt with things that feel troublesome is to plan for them, not to stay away from them. That is the reason, for this Dry January particularly, preparation is critical. Remind yourself why you are doing this, make a rundown and take a gander at it when hard times arise. Dispose of any alcohol in your home – if it is not there, you cannot be tempted. Arrange for what you will do if cravings strike.

Assuming January 2021 brings us some awful news, further anxiety, or stress, what are you going to do? Are there ways you can loosen up that do not include alcohol? Settle on your ways of dealing with stress early so you are prepared.

2. TAKE CARE OF YOUR OVERALL MENTAL HEALTH.

Any change is superior to no change. Amid stress, we can wind up drinking even more frequently or more intensely. To ensure you are less tempted to go after a drink to help you cope, take care of your overall mental health. Ensure you eat healthily, take breaks from the news occasionally, and get outside once every day if possible. Abstaining from drinking will help you work out healthier coping mechanisms for the difficult feelings you are experiencing.

3. DISCOVER ALTERNATIVE TREATS AND WAYS TO RELAX

I have changed how I associate with friends, rather than meeting in the bar with drinks (or a virtual catch up with cocktails), I have asked if we could meet for a walk. It fortifies the help when friends consent to plan something other than what's expected for help with you being alcohol-free, in addition to the fresh air is greatly better!"

CARMEL

My best counsel is to attempt alternatives, for example, alcohol-free beer, botanicals with tonic or other mixers."

COLLEEN

Alcohol maybe your go-to treat when you need to unwind, or when you believe you merit a reward. To make your Dry January simpler, take a stab at finding different things to treat yourself with to break the relationship between treating, unwinding, and alcohol. Ease yourself into it by requesting some alcohol-free drinks or some fancy soft drinks or teas, for instance, so you have them close by toward the end of a long working day.

4. BE GENTLE WITH YOURSELF

Do whatever it takes not to zero in on the thing you are losing, but rather the thing you are adding to your life. Add loads of new things to try out - strolls, a hobby, new foods, new chocolate! Surrendering alcohol is enriching.

I would state perhaps attempt to consider what it is you truly look for from a drink. Is it a sense of belonging? Association with friends? Rest and unwinding? Alcohol guarantees a lot, however, does not generally convey any of those things. Truly, it tastes decent (some of it does) yet so does loads of things! Prepare a cake instead!

One of the key things we need you to recollect this Dry January is to be gentle with yourself. We have all experienced a great deal this past year, so do not feel crippled when change does not come as effectively as you had expected. You can do this, and we are right by your side.

Difficulties are an ordinary, yet baffling, part of changing a propensity. But on the other hand, they are an extraordinary open door for learning and pushing ahead emphatically.

My new vastly diminished drinking design was hit hard by CONVID-19. My arrangements to proceed onward with my life were marked by the first lockdown... I have been drinking most nights since lockdown – but I have figured out how to hold my drinking down to adjust and about safe drinking levels... I will be thoughtful with myself. I

t was an intense year, I returned a touch, but I will refocus with

Dry January. I participated in Dry January 2020 and felt a ton of advantages from it. Be that as it may, at that point lockdown occurred, and she fell back into behavior patterns she would preferably break. With the assistance of Dry January, ending those propensities is what I intend to do!

CHAPTER FOUR

A GUIDE TO SEX
AND DATING
DURING DRY JANUARY

Regardless of whether you are not participating in Dry January, you presumably know somebody who is. Surrendering alcohol for a whole month following the festive abundance of December has become an undeniably common New Year health kick. Indeed, one out of five Americans said they were attempting the less booze test in the previous year (however it is untold who made it the full 31 days).

It is not interesting to sort out precisely why Dry January has gotten so famous. Those keeping away from alcohol are bound to save money, sleep better, and appreciate a variety of health and wellness benefits like improved skin and reduced blood pressure. In case you are a regular drinker, you will likewise give your liver a well-deserved break.

All that stated, while Dry January might be admirable, it is additionally highly challenging — particularly in case you are expecting to remain active on the dating scene. Dating in January can be overwhelming for individuals undertaking the Dry January challenge, House of Ardent's sex and relationships expert Lianne Young. What do you drink when you are out on a date if it is not something to help loosen up your nerves?

Notwithstanding, Young calls attention to that while alcoholic drinks might assist with nerves, they should never be permitted to turn into a brace or personality substitution.

It is acceptable to become more acquainted with somebody sober since that way you become more acquainted with the real them, and that is truly what is significant, she adds.

Given this current in mind, here is a manual for dating during Dry January that will ideally eliminate any pre-meetup anxiety realizing alcohol will not be in play.

1. IT IS FINE TO FEEL SOMEWHAT NERVOUS

Being anxious before a date is typical, says Dru Jaeger, co-author of How to Be a Mindful Drinker: Cut Down, Stop For a Bit, or Quit, a guide to help moderate your drinking propensities. It is enticing to attempt to conceal those nerves with a drink, however, it is a no-nonsense fix. It is smarter to recognize your nerves and afterward focus on the other individual.

Jaeger says this methodology has two clear advantages: It will distract you from feeling apprehensive, and it will most likely cause your date to feel great that you are giving them so much attention.

2. BE FORTHRIGHT ABOUT THE REALITY YOU'RE DOING DRY JANUARY

Assuming going on dates that involve alcohol, you might feel self-conscious about telling your date that you will not drink. All things considered, there is a lingering disgrace around being teetotal that might make you worry you will put on a show of being exhausting without a beer in your hand. Whatever you do, do not allow this to play at the forefront of your thoughts.

It might feel like a serious deal for you, but [you are not drinking] is simply one more reality about you for them, notes Jaeger. If they respond badly, do not worry about it. You would not have any desire to date somebody who does not support your decisions at any rate.

3. EXPAND YOUR CONCEPT OF WHAT A DATE SHOULD BE

an obvious option in contrast to meeting for drinks. Convening for coffee instead. Coffee dates are extraordinary in case you are hoping to build a long-term relationship since they are increasingly slow engrossing, says Young.

Nonetheless, Young surrenders that coffee dates tend to turn somewhat bland over time, recommending utilizing your innovative side when considering how to become more acquainted with each other.

Recollect that dates do not need to be hours long, and they do not need to be at night, states Jaeger, who suggests an excursion to a gallery or a stroll in the recreation center as relaxing alternatives and roller-skating or rock climbing as more energetic ones. However, the alternatives are as interminable as your imagination.

When you get past the possibility that dating needs to include drinking, you might think that it turns into an even more invigorating and compensating process. Regardless of whether there is no romantic spark between you and your date, you will have shared an advancing beneficial experience.

4. Should You End Up At A Bar Anyway, Mocktails Can Be Your Friend.

Exemplary cocktails without the booze have progressed significantly since your parents would get you a Shirley Temple on family holidays. Request that your bartender to stir up something astonishing and alcohol-free, and they will almost certainly oblige.

5. REMEMBER THE BENEFICIAL OUTCOMES THAT ACCOMPANY SOBER DATING

The principal advantage of sober dating is that you will recall your date says, Jaeger. Regardless of whether it goes splendidly, horribly, or undoubtedly somewhere in between, you can be certain that you remained in charge, introduced your best self, and we are truly ready to focus on the individual you date.

You are likewise bound to know without a doubt whether you need to see that individual once more, which is urgent to dating effectively and successfully.

Also, you have known about an easily overlooked detail called whiskey d*CK, correct? Indeed, even the incomparable William Shakespeare rather adorably alluded to alcohol's negative impact on our sexual undertakings as brewer's hang. It merits recalling that another feature of dating without alcohol during Dry January could be more adventurous and engaging sex (that you recollect, as well)

WHAT DOES THE EXPERT SAY?

Lifestyle, relationships, and sex guru, Lianne Young, tells United Kingdom's highest-circulation print newspaper called metro that 'Individuals drink for a variety of reasons, ordinarily for confidence and freedom during the honeymoon period. Individuals drink when they celebrate, embrace, and become acquainted with someone – particularly the opposite sex. Unfortunately, sometimes individuals additionally end up falling into bed, and some vibe awful about it in the morning. 'Keep in mind, alcohol gives us confidence and the boldness to do things we, in any case, wouldn't do.

It can likewise suppress emotions and abrogate our typical defense mechanism. 'Coffee dates are incredible in case you're hoping to build a long- term relationship; it is slower, additionally absorbing and you will have no second thoughts, and obviously, you can leave in case you're not happy with your date.

'Notwithstanding, coffee can be boring, and I do not figure it will assume control over dating as another pattern instead of alcohol – Dry January is essentially Dry January and put pressure on individuals to quit for only one month, as opposed to the individual wanting to quit any pretense of drinking.

'What individuals ought to do as an alternative to drunken dating is to arrange dates with smaller surroundings of individuals drinking. 'My recommendations would be to go to dinner or cooking. If you are dating and alcohol is a major part of it, and you have feelings for your date, at that point, I suggest organizing a daytime date. This way you have real feelings and actions, and can talk about the following dates, what you like doing, and perhaps what you can do together. 'Try not to put resources into a relationship which is built exclusively around a pub, it won't work. Rather choose what you need for yourself long-term.'

CHAPTER FIVE

Post Dry January: 5 Tips To Make The Most Of Life Alcohol-Free

I began my journey to alcohol-free doing Dry January in 2015, and while there have been many good and bad times en route I am presently carrying on with life joyfully without alcohol.

Claiming you are contemplating broadening your alcohol-free period for a couple of months, or perhaps a lifetime, you are not alone! Although it may feel like it sometimes, taking a break from boozing or living life AF(Alcohol-Free) is getting progressively famous. Let assume you are anticipating prolonging your Dry January streak or have chosen to live a long term without alcohol, read on for the 5 tips on making the most out of your time alcohol-free.

POST DRY JANUARY, GET COMFORTABLE WITH YOUR DECISION NOT TO DRINK

For what reason would you say you are extending your alcohol-free period beyond Dry January or choosing to live life alcohol-free? Would you like to lose weight? Save Money? Be more productive? Set aside an effort to consider why you need to keep experiencing life alcohol-free and write it down to remain on target when your motivation fades. Documenting how much money you are saving and the amount you are (not) drinking through the Dry January app is additionally an extraordinary method to remain inspired and perceive how much cash (and calories) you have saved through not drinking.

DO NOT AVOID THE PUB (OR GET-TOGETHERS)

Except if you want to that is! Try not to feel like not drinking implies you need to remain at home forevermore. Capitalize on get-togethers, and the pub, by choosing what you must drink beforehand and returning home when it gets exhausting. Remind yourself why you have chosen to extend your Dry January challenge before going out for additional inspiration.

MAKE THE MOST OF HANGOVER-FREE MORNINGS

What do you love to do however frequently do not have time for? Invest significant time in the morning to accomplish something you appreciate doing – like going for a run, investing time with your children, or having a comfortable breakfast – to take advantage of the time you may have recently spent hungover or in bed.

EMBRACE COMMUNITY

You are not by any means the only one not drinking. Allow me to say that once more. You are not by any means the only one not drinking! It might feel like it when you are out with your friends but lots of individuals are attempting life alcohol-free and getting a charge out of the advantages that accompany it. Social media (love it or disdain it) implies you can connect with people across the world and there are some incredible online networks you can engage in; I recommend Club soda for lots of likeminded supportive folks.

Think Of Drinking (And Not Drinking) Does Not Define You.

Drinking, or not drinking, is just one small part of your life and your decisions. You are still you, with or without the alcohol. Your choice not to drink might be the solitary thing people seem to talk to you about for the first few week's post January however they will get bored of asking you and you will become accustomed to it! Zero in on all the stuff you are doing, the entirety of the pleasant you are having, and the things that make you extraordinary and keep going however long it feels right for you.